I0830852

WEIGHT LOSS ONLY

The Simplified guide for sustainable weight loss

By

Richard L. Patton

Copyright © by Richard L. Patton 2023. All rights reserved.

Before this document is duplicated or reproduced in any manner, the publisher's consent must be gained. Therefore, the contents within can neither be stored electronically, transferred nor kept in a database. Neither in Part nor full can the document be copied, scanned, faxed or retained without approval from the publisher or creator.

Table of Contents

INTRODUCTION 4

CHAPTER 1........................8

Factors That Cause Weight Gain..8

CHAPTER 2 42

Some Hard Truths About Weight Loss.......................42

CHAPTER 3.........................58

Simple Strategies To Prevent Weight Gain........................58

CHAPTER 4.......................117

Foods That Burn Fat and Rev Up Your Metabolism..........117

INTRODUCTION

A loose connective tissue made primarily of adipocytes is known as adipose tissue, body fat, or simply fat (Fats cells).

Increased bodily weight is referred to as weight gain. This might be brought on by a rise in muscle mass, fat deposition, an abundance of fluids like water, or other elements. One sign of a significant medical problem is weight gain.

When more energy (as calories from food and drink consumption) is obtained than is burned during daily activities, such as regular physiological processes and physical activity, weight gain results.

One may become overweight or obese, which is commonly described as having more body fat (adipose tissue) than is thought to be healthy if enough weight is acquired as a result of increasing body fat deposits. The Body Mass

Index (BMI) calculates the ideal, inadequate, and excessive weight based on the ratio of body weight to height.

Excess adipose tissue (fat) is a frequent problem, particularly in areas with copious food sources and sedentary lifestyles.

Obesity and overweight may raise the chance of developing several illnesses, including diabetes, heart disease, and some types of cancer, as well as short- and long-term health issues when pregnant.

CHAPTER 1

FACTORS THAT CAUSE WEIGHT GAIN

Many appear to believe that a lack of willpower is what leads to weight gain and obesity.

That's not accurate. Even while eating habits and lifestyle choices account for the majority of weight gain, some people have difficulty in this area.

The problem is that a variety of biological aspects, including hormones and heredity, contribute to overeating. Some folks just tend to acquire weight.

Yes, people may change their lifestyle and behavior to compensate for hereditary disadvantages. Willpower, commitment, and persistence are needed to make a lifestyle change.

However, it is oversimplified to assert that conduct is solely a product of willpower.

They don't consider all the other elements that eventually influence people's actions and timing.

Here are some variables, many of which have nothing to do with willpower, that are major contributors to weight gain and even obesity

1. Food Accessibility

Food availability, which has expanded significantly over the past several centuries, is another element that has a significant impact on people's waistlines.

Food, especially fast food, is widely available today. In stores, appealing items are displayed in areas where you are most likely to see them.

Another issue is that, especially in America, unhealthy, whole meals are frequently more affordable.

Some folks, especially those who live in less affluent areas, don't even have access to actual food options like fresh fruits and vegetables.

These communities exclusively have convenience stores that offer beverages, candies, and processed packaged junk food.

If there is no choice, how can it be a question of choice?

Finding fresh, healthful meals may be challenging or pricey in some places, forcing individuals to purchase unhealthy junk food as their only option.

2. Food Dependence

The reward regions in your brain are stimulated by a variety of high-fat, sugar-sweetened junk meals.

These meals are frequently contrasted with substances that are frequently misused, such as alcohol, cocaine, nicotine, and cannabis.

Junk food addiction can develop in those who are vulnerable. Similar to how those who struggle with alcohol addiction lose control over their drinking, these people also lose control over their eating.

Addiction is a complicated problem that may be very hard to resolve. You lose your ability to make independent decisions when you get addicted to anything, and your brain's biochemistry takes over.

Some people have significant addictions to or appetites for eating. This is particularly true of junk meals heavy in fat and sugar that activate the brain's reward centers.

3. Violent Marketing

Marketers for manufacturers of junk food are quite aggressive.

Sometimes they try to

promote extremely harmful items as healthy ones, which is an unethical technique.

These businesses also make false statements. Even worse, they intentionally target youngsters with their marketing.

Children are becoming obese, diabetic, and hooked to junk food in modern society before they are mature enough to make these kinds of decisions for themselves.

Food companies spend a lot of money advertising junk food, sometimes particularly aiming it toward kids who lack the maturity and experience to recognize when they are being deceived.

4. Artificial junk foods

Foods that have undergone extensive processing typically only include refined components and additives.

These goods are made to be inexpensive, durable, and difficult to resist due to their incredible flavor.

Food producers aim to boost sales by making products as delicious as possible. However, they also encourage overeating.

Today's processed foods tend to have very little in common with whole foods. These items are carefully crafted and made to hook consumers.

Processed foods are abundant in stores and are difficult to avoid. Additionally, these goods encourage overeating.

5. Insulin

One of the many things that insulin controls is how much energy is stored. Its job includes instructing fat cells to store fat and retain any fat they currently contain.

Many overweight and obese people's Western diets encourage insulin resistance. As a result, the body's insulin levels rise throughout, causing energy to be stored in fat cells as opposed to being used.

Although there is debate regarding insulin's relationship to obesity, research point to a direct relationship between elevated insulin levels and the emergence of obesity.

Reducing your diet to simple or refined carbs while increasing your intake of fiber is one of the greatest methods to reduce your insulin.

Without the need for portion control or calorie tracking, this typically results in a spontaneous decrease in caloric intake and uncomplicated weight loss.

The development of obesity is associated with high insulin

levels and insulin resistance. Reduce your diet of refined carbohydrates and increase your fiber intake to lower your insulin levels.

6. Certain Drugs

As a side effect, several medicinal medicines might make you gain weight.

For instance, antidepressants have been associated with gradual weight gain.

Antipsychotic drugs and medications for diabetes are more examples.

These medications do not weaken your willpower. They change how your body and brain work, slowing down or speeding up your metabolism.

In conclusion, several drugs may cause weight gain by lowering calorie expenditure or boosting hunger.

7. Resistance To Leptin

Another hormone that has a

significant impact on obesity is leptin. It is generated by fat cells, and as fat mass increases, blood levels rise. Leptin levels are hence particularly high in obese individuals.

High leptin levels are associated with decreased appetite in healthy individuals. It should communicate to your brain how much fat you have when it's functioning properly.

Leptin is not functioning

properly in many obese persons because, for unknown reasons, it cannot penetrate the blood-brain barrier.

Leptin resistance is a condition that is thought to be a major contributor to the pathophysiology of obesity.

In many obese people, leptin—a hormone that decreases appetite—does not function.

8. Genetics

There is a large hereditary component to obesity. Compared to children of lean parents, children of obese parents are significantly more likely to be obese.

This does not imply that obesity is entirely inevitable. Which genes are expressed and which are not can be greatly influenced by what you consume.

When non-industrialized countries adopt a normal

Western diet, obesity rates
rise quickly in those societies.
Their environment and the
signals it delivered to their
genes altered them more
than their genes did.

The fact that obesity and
being overweight often run in
families suggests that genes
may be involved. If one or
both of your parents are
obese or overweight, your
chances of getting
overweight are higher.

The quantity of body fat you

retain and the locations of that additional fat may be influenced by your genes.

Simply put, genetic factors do influence your propensity to gain weight. This is very well illustrated by studies on identical twins

Some individuals seem to have a hereditary predisposition to weight growth and obesity.

9. Sugar

The worst element of the contemporary diet could be added sugar.

That's because consuming too much sugar alters your body's biochemistry and hormones. In turn, this results in a weight increase.

Half of the added sugar is glucose and half is fructose. Starches and other foods can provide people with glucose, but the bulk of fructose comes from added sugar.

Increased insulin levels and insulin resistance may result

from consuming too much sugar. Additionally, it does not stimulate satiety the same way that glucose does.

Sugar causes more energy to be stored in the body, which ultimately leads to obesity.

According to scientists, consuming too much sugar may be one of the primary causes of obesity.

10. Ethnicity Or Race

There are several racial and

ethnic minority groups where obesity is more prevalent. African Americans have the greatest rates of obesity among American adults, followed by Hispanics/Latinos and finally Caucasians.

Both men and women may agree on this. Despite having the lowest rates of obesity among men and women, Asian Americans are nonetheless susceptible to illnesses linked to obesity if they have a lot of unhealthy abdominal fat, even if their body mass index (BMI) is lower.

11. Age

As people age, many of them put on weight. Adults with a normal BMI frequently begin gaining weight in their early 20s and keep adding pounds until they are 60 to 65 years old. Children who are obese are also more prone to become obese adults.

12. False Information

People are ignorant about diet and health all around the world.

There are several causes for this, but the issue is mostly influenced by the sources of information that individuals use.

For instance, a lot of websites disseminate false or outright misleading advice regarding diet and health.

The findings of scientific

research are regularly taken out of context in some news outlets, and they are sometimes oversimplified or misinterpreted.

Some material may simply be out-of-date or based on unproven hypotheses.

As well, food businesses are involved. Some advertise useless things, like weight loss pills.

Strategies for losing weight

that is based on erroneous information might impede your success. It's crucial to make wise source selections.

Inaccurate information may play a role in some persons gaining weight. It could also make losing weight more challenging.

13. Sex

In the US, black or Hispanic women are more likely to be obese than their male counterparts. Where the body stores fat may also depend on a person's sex. In women, the hips and buttocks frequently swell with fat.

Typically, males get belly or abdominal fat. Even if a person has a normal weight, excess fat, especially if it is around the belly, might increase their chance of developing health issues.

14. Location

Your diet and exercise habits, as well as your availability of nutritious foods and active places to go, may be influenced by where you live, work, play, and go to church.

For instance, having a lot of grocery stores nearby can enhance your access to higher-quality, lower-calorie items. You could be inspired to be more physically active if you live in a community with lots of green spaces and places where you can safely engage in physical exercise.

It could also be simpler for you to consume unhealthily unhealthy, high-calorie foods where you work and pray. You might not find healthier, lower-calorie alternatives in the vending machines, cafeterias, or special events at your place of employment or place of worship. Pick the healthier selections whenever you can, and keep your sweets to a tiny piece of pie or cake.

15. Customs And Culture Of The Family

Your weight and health may be impacted by your family's food and lifestyle choices. At family gatherings, some families could eat a lot of unhealthy food or drinks that are heavy in fat, salt, and added sugars. Additionally, some families may spend a lot of time passively engaging in activities like watching TV, using a computer, or using a mobile device.

Due to common eating and lifestyle practices, your social, ethnic, or religious group culture may also have an impact on your weight and health. Foods and beverages with a lot of fat, salt, and added sugars may be popular in some cultures.

Some typical meal preparation techniques, including frying, may result in a large consumption of calories. Over time, eating meals that are often heavy in calories, fat, and sugar may cause weight gain.

16. Inadequate Slumber

Lack of sleep can lead to increased calorie intake and snacking. Adults should sleep for 7 to 9 hours per night if they are between the ages of 18 and 64, and for 7 to 8 hours if they are 65 or older.

CHAPTER 2

SOME HARD TRUTHS ABOUT WEIGHT LOSS

1. Your Body Opposes You.

It's not only in your head: When you strive to lose weight, your body is a battleground in addition to your appetites. According to Australian experts, losing weight causes the hormones ghrelin, which promotes appetite, to increase, and leptin, which tells your brain that you're full, to drop.

According to the study, this hormonal imbalance persists even after you achieve weight reduction, making it much more difficult for you to keep the pounds off.

Plus, your metabolism will slow down if you eliminate calories too soon.

If you substantially reduce your caloric intake and lose a lot of weight rapidly, you may be also losing some muscle. Since muscle serves as the metabolic engine, losing muscle slows down metabolism. Because you were restricting yourself for such a long time, eating too little also increases your likelihood of rebounding and moving oppositely by overeating.

We suggest acting more moderately: It has been demonstrated that the best long-term weight loss strategies involve increasing physical activity and reducing calorie intake.

2. There Are No Easy Solutions

There are no magic medicines or magical cures that can make you lose 30 pounds in time for your high school reunion next month; wishing it would happen won't make it happen either. It's challenging to remain patient when attempting to reduce weight.

But resist the urge to take a risk and try something novel. Fast starvation diets can mess with your metabolism, which can harm your long-term attempts to lose weight. Keep in mind that one to two pounds of weight reduction every week is the simplest to sustain when you begin your diet.

3. Exercise Can't Win Everything

Yes, exercise aids in weight loss and weight maintenance; according to a National Weight Control Registry report, persons who maintain their weight reduction exercise for at least 60 minutes most days. However, it's extremely difficult to reduce weight alone via exercise.

Do the math, please: 369 calories are burned during 60 minutes of 12-mph riding by a 135-pound individual. All you need is a protein bar after your workout to gain it all back.

You can understand how challenging it is to work out your way through a bad diet when you consider that you must burn 3,500 more calories per day than you take in to lose one pound of fat. Instead, you must exercise and control what you consume. If dieting has any "magic," it's in that combo.

4. Supplements for Diet Don't Work

Though enticing, there is little proof that the little medicines that boost metabolism help. The use of liquid diets, fad diets, and over-the-counter diet pills was not associated with weight reduction.

So what did work? reducing

dietary fat, increasing exercise, using prescription weight-loss drugs, and enrolling in for-profit weight-loss programs.

5. Fad Diets That Don't Last Long

Grapefruit. maple sugar. Cabbage. Apple cider vinegar Juice. All of these "magic" diets promise to make you lose weight and start burning fat.

The unpleasant truth: Calorie restriction makes fad diets

effective in the short term, but they don't provide effects that persist.

The issue is that most people lack the will to completely avoid certain food categories or drastically reduce their calorie consumption, which leads to a return to a more calorically rich, inclusive diet over time.

6. One Diet Does Not Apply to All

The diet that works for your friend, coworker, mother, or sister could not work for you since every person's body is different.

When determining the ideal weight loss strategy, take into account your age, gender, level of exercise, metabolism, age, and family medical history.

If you don't allow yourself to eat any of the things you like when you're dieting, Jo advises, you'll feel deprived and be less inclined to follow a general healthy eating plan.

To lose weight successfully, customize your diet to your needs and realize that no one diet will be effective for everyone.

7. Cardio Exercise Is Vital (and Strength Training Helps Too)

Adults should engage in at least two days of muscle-strengthening activities each week in addition to 150 minutes of moderate-intensity aerobic exercise or 75 minutes of vigorous aerobic activity (or a combination of both), per the 2018 Physical Activity Guidelines for Americans, which were published in November 2018 in the Journal of the American Medical Association. Every little amount matters, thus it's advised to exercise more throughout the day, even if it's only taking a short stroll around the block.

Most people should be able to reduce weight using these suggestions. However, those who are obese or need to shed a lot of weight need to be even more active, gradually increasing their daily activity to at least 30 minutes.

Don't neglect strength training either, advises Jo, since it helps to maintain the joint health and functionality required for all that cardio.

Having additional muscle mass also slightly speeds up your metabolism and improves your appearance.

8. He Can Consume More Food Than She Can

Men can eat more than women and yet lose weight, which doesn't seem fair. Because of their greater size, the muscular mass, and higher amounts of the hormone testosterone, which stimulates muscle growth, males often burn more calories naturally than women.

Additionally, because males do not need to store the energy necessary to have children, the male body is genetically programmed to have greater muscle and less fat than the female body.

The scale will appreciate you once you accept this reality and start eating less than your male partner or pals.

9. It's Not a Diet, It's a Change in Lifestyle

You must alter your behavior throughout the months and years after you achieve your desired weight if you want to lose weight and keep it off.

That's because after you end

your "diet," you'll probably put the weight back on that you're worked so hard to lose.

Making permanent lifestyle adjustments, such as choosing nutritious foods virtually every meal and engaging in a significant amount of activity each week, are necessary for weight reduction success.

CHAPTER 3

SIMPLE STRATEGIES TO PREVENT WEIGHT GAIN

Making dietary modifications, such as consuming more protein and fewer refined carbohydrates, may accelerate fat reduction over time and improve your health in general.

It can be difficult to lose body fat; it frequently calls for perseverance, hard work, and devotion.

The most efficient strategy to achieve and maintain a healthy weight is to change your food, lifestyle, and exercise regimen, although many fad diets and fat-burning products claim instant results.

You may also encourage sustained, long-term weight loss by taking a few easy actions, which will also benefit your general health.

Here are the few methods for

accelerating fat reduction;

1. Consume A Lot Of Protein

Consuming more protein-rich meals may help you eat less and burn more calories.

Several studies have linked eating more high-quality protein with a decreased risk of obesity and extra body fat.

According to another study, a high-protein diet may aid in maintaining metabolism and muscle mass while losing weight.

Increasing your protein consumption may also result in greater feelings of satiety, less appetite, and lower calorie intake, all of which promote weight reduction.

High-quality protein diets can aid in weight loss by encouraging satiation (the sensation of fullness), assisting in maintaining muscle mass while doing so and boosting diet-induced thermogenesis (the burning of calories from digestion).

Consuming protein can also lessen your cravings for sugar and carbs by reducing the release of the hunger hormone ghrelin.

According to one study, raising a person's protein intake to 25% of daily calories helped reduce the desire for late-night snacks in half and decreased cravings overall by 60%.

More protein in your diet may also aid increase metabolism,

increasing the number of calories your body burns during the day.

Consider including a couple of servings of high-protein foods each day in your diet. Meat, fish, eggs, beans, tofu, and dairy items like milk, cheese, and yogurt are examples of foods high in protein.

A decreased risk of abdominal fat may be linked to eating more protein. Additionally, it could reduce hunger, consume fewer calories, and maintain muscle mass.

2. Sleep More

One easy way to achieve and maintain a healthy weight is to go to bed a little earlier or sleep in a little later.

Several studies link losing weight to getting enough sleep.

One 10-year research found an increased risk of obesity in young women who slept fewer than 6 hours per night.

Another small research found that, as compared to a control group, participants on a low-calorie diet lost less fat when they slept 1 hour less each night.

According to another study, sleep deprivation may be linked to changes in hunger hormones, increased appetite, and a higher risk of obesity.

According to research, persons who sleep for fewer than seven hours in 24 hours are more likely to be obese than those who routinely receive at least seven hours.

Sleep is crucial for shedding pounds and building strength. Leptin and ghrelin, the two hormones that control hunger, are interfered with by sleep loss, increasing the likelihood that you may engage in unhealthy eating behaviors.

Another hormone that increases when you don't get enough sleep is cortisol. Additionally, the body releases it in reaction to stress, and it plays a significant role in the buildup of belly fat.

Feel free to use your aim to reduce body fat percentage as an excuse to go to bed earlier because the typical adult only gets six hours of sleep or less.

Sleeping off the pounds is the

simplest approach to reducing weight.

Even though everyone has different sleep demands, most studies have found that getting at least 7 hours of sleep each night has the greatest positive effects on both weight control and general health.

Maintain a regular sleep schedule, cut back on your evening coffee intake, and avoid using electronics just before bed to encourage a healthy sleep cycle.

Getting adequate sleep may help you eat less, feel less hungry, and minimize your chance of gaining weight.

4. Commence Your Strength Training

Muscles are worked against resistance during a strength-training workout. Over time, it promotes strength and muscular mass, and it typically entails lifting weights.

Research shows that strength training has a variety of positive effects on health, particularly in terms of fat reduction.

In addition to reducing visceral fat, which is a form of fat that surrounds your internal organs in your abdomen, resistance exercise may also drastically reduce body fat mass.

Another study found that 5 months of strength training

was superior to aerobic exercise alone in lowering body fat in obese teenagers.

Additionally, resistance exercise could maintain lean mass, which could boost your body's resting metabolic rate.

Exercise is equally as important for fat loss as diet. You should start lifting weights if you want to maximize fat reduction.

The greatest notable decreases in fat mass occur when you mix diet and strength training, when comparing diet alone to diet plus resistance exercise. You'll also seem toned more quickly if you increase your lean muscle mass while decreasing your fat mass.

Consider seeking the advice of a personal trainer if you're learning how to include resistance training in your workout program for the first time.

While adults should engage in strength-training exercises that target all main muscle groups (the legs, hips, back, belly, chest, shoulders, and arms) at least twice a week, according to general guidelines from the Centers for Disease Control and Prevention (CDC).

In contrast to a control group, strength training increased people's resting metabolic rates, whereas aerobic exercise had no metabolic impact.

A few simple strategies to begin strength training include using gym equipment, lifting weights, and bodyweight exercises.

Strength exercise may not only help you lose body fat but also target belly fat and raise resting energy expenditure.

5. Consume More Beneficial Fats

Increasing your consumption of good fats may prevent weight gain, even though this may seem paradoxical.

In comparison to a low-fat diet, 12-month research found that adopting a Mediterranean diet high in good fats from nuts and olive oil led to higher long-term weight loss.

Another study found that when compared to diets lacking olive oil, meals rich in olive oil led to significant decreases in body weight and belly fat.

Trans fats, a kind of fat that is frequently found in fried or processed meals, are also linked to greater long-term weight gain.

Focus on consuming healthy "good" fats like polyunsaturated fats and reducing damaging "bad" fats like trans fats rather than following a low-fat diet.

Eating fat makes you feel fuller after meals and slows down digestion, which makes it easier to lose weight.

Consume fish, avocados, olives and olive oil, eggs, nuts and nut butter, seeds, dark chocolate, and other foods high in heart-healthy monounsaturated and polyunsaturated fats.

Trans fats, which are included in fried meals, vegetable shortening, margarine, baked products, and processed snack items, should be avoided in the interim.

Avocados, nuts, seeds, avocado oil, olive oil, coconut

oil, and avocados are just a few examples of healthy fats.

It's vital to manage your consumption of healthy fat because it still contains a lot of calories.

Try replacing fried meals, processed products, and refined oils with healthier alternatives instead of eating more fat overall.

A decreased risk of weight gain is linked to a larger consumption of healthy fats like olive oil and almonds.

6. Be Cautious When Drinking

One of the simplest methods to encourage long-term, sustained fat reduction is to swap out sugary drinks with healthy options.

For instance, drinks like soda that have been sweetened with sugar are frequently high in calories and low in nutrients. Alcohol has a lot of calories and might make you less inhibited, which can make you more likely to overeat.

According to a recent study, ultra-processed foods (UPPs) make up about 70% of the average American's diet starting at age 5, which is bad news for body fat.

UPPs are incredibly high in bad fats, which makes them highly tasty and addicting. These unhealthy fats are frequently combined with additional sugars and salt in scandalous quantities.

Additionally, people frequently consume excessive amounts of highly processed, nutrient-poor, prepackaged items like cookies, bagels, chips, and margarine.

The 152 pounds of refined sugar consumed annually by the average American may seriously interfere with blood sugar levels and raise insulin levels, which can have an impact on fat storage.

Refined sugars, which are common in highly processed goods, are empty calories. Reduced calorie intake encourages the body to burn stored fat, which lowers the body's overall fat percentage.

Up to 30% of a person's daily caloric consumption can come from high-calorie beverages like soda, wine, and other sweetened liquids. These beverages frequently include high-fructose corn syrup, which has been related to fatty liver disease and other illnesses in humans.

Drink extra water instead. Because they are too busy, forget, or don't keep track of it, more than half of American people don't drink enough water.

Water consumption is crucial for burning off both stored fat and fat from meals and drinks. A study published in Frontiers in Nutrition indicated that drinking more water enhanced lipolysis, or the breakdown of fat, and decreased the formation of new fat.

How much water does one need? The general recommendation is to consume half your body weight in ounces each day. So aim to drink 75 ounces of water every day if you weigh 150 pounds.

Alcohol use and sugar-sweetened beverage consumption have both been linked in studies to an increased risk of abdominal fat.

Choose calorie-free drinks like water or green tea instead.

Drinking 1 pint (570 mL) of water before a meal boosted feelings of fullness, lowered appetite, and reduced the number of calories consumed during the meal, according to small research involving 14 young males.

As an alternative, green tea has both caffeine and a lot of antioxidants, which may aid

to speed up metabolism and
fat burning.

Drinks with added sugar and
alcoholic beverages may
raise the risk of belly fat.

Change them out for green
tea or water, which have been
found to accelerate fat and
weight reduction.

7. Eat Plenty Of Fiber

Plant foods include soluble
fiber, which absorbs water
and passes slowly through

your digestive system to help you feel fuller for longer.

Increasing your consumption of foods high in fiber may prevent weight gain, according to research. Fruits, vegetables, legumes, whole grains, nuts, and seeds are some examples of these foods.

For instance, 345-person research found a link between enhanced dietary adherence and higher weight reduction when consuming more fiber.

Compared to sugars, protein, and carbs, fiber makes you feel fuller and takes longer to digest.

According to research, those who followed a diet with no extra dietary restrictions and ingested 30 grams of fiber daily lost a considerable amount of weight.

Eating foods like oats, legumes, fruits, beans, and wheat bran as dietary sources of fiber since they are "in addition to weight reduction, heart-healthy, excellent for gut health, and can lower risk of diabetes and some cancers."

Additionally, studies show that fiber is effective at getting rid of stubborn belly fat, which is crucial because belly fat is associated with many extra health problems, such as an increased risk of type 2 diabetes and cardiovascular disease.

Independent of calorie consumption, a different

evaluation indicated that increasing soluble fiber intake significantly reduced body weight and belly fat.

Increasing your intake of fiber by eating more fresh fruits, vegetables, and legumes may help you feel fuller for longer and lose weight.

8. Opt For Whole Grains Rather Than Processed Carbohydrates

You may be able to shed additional body fat by reducing your diet of refined carbohydrates.

Refined grains lose their bran and germ during processing, leaving behind a finished good that is deficient in fiber and minerals.

Additionally, refined carbohydrates frequently have a high glycemic index (GI), which may result in blood sugar rises and crashes that stimulate appetite.

However, if you consume refined carbohydrates on their own as opposed to as a component of a balanced diet, you're more likely to experience these side effects.

Furthermore, studies link long-term belly fat accumulation to diets heavy in refined carbohydrates. A diet rich in whole grains, on the other hand, is associated with a lower body mass index (BMI), lower weight, and a smaller waist circumference.

Just remember that conventional weight measurements like BMI don't accurately depict a person's overall health.

Aim to substitute healthy grains like whole wheat, quinoa, buckwheat, barley, and oats for refined carbohydrates found in pastries, processed meals, pasta, white bread, and morning cereals.

Whole grains are optimal for long-term, sustained fat loss since refined carbohydrates are deficient in fiber and minerals.

9. Increase Aerobic Activity

One of the most popular types of exercise is cardio, commonly referred to as aerobic exercise. It refers to any form of exercise that focuses on strengthening the heart and lungs.

The best strategy to increase fat burning and weight reduction may be to include exercise in your program.

For instance, a study of 15 research found a link between middle-aged women's increased aerobic activity and lower abdominal fat.

Exercises that burn calories continuously, such as cycling, jogging, and walking, are categorized as cardiovascular workouts. They both increase metabolism and aid in effective calorie burning.

Calculate your maximal heart rate by deducting your age from 220 to get the most out of your fat-burning cardio routines.

The heart rate range that appears to be most beneficial for burning fat is between 70% and 80% of that value. The ideal quantity of cardio for fat loss will vary from person to person, just like many other factors discussed here.

However, the overall CDC recommendations call for 150 minutes or more of moderate-intensity aerobic exercise per week.

Consider combining high-intensity interval training (HIIT) with your exercise routine if you want to accelerate your fat reduction.

In HIIT, short bursts of high-intensity exercise are interspersed with rest periods or intervals of lower-intensity exercise.

According to studies, this exercise technique can reduce body fat by 28.5% more than steady-state aerobic exercises like power walking.

According to other research, aerobic exercise may enhance muscle mass while reducing body fat, belly fat, and waist circumference.

The majority of research suggests 150–300 minutes of "moderate–intensity" exercise per week, which translates to 20–40 minutes of cardio each day.

Cardio exercises include walking, cycling, swimming, and running, to name a few.

According to studies, people tend to shed more body fat when they engage in greater aerobic activity. Exercise may also help build muscle and lower waist size.

10. Consume Coffee

Coffee contains caffeine, which stimulates the central nervous system, raises metabolism, and speeds up fatty acid breakdown.

Additionally, it has been demonstrated that caffeine increases fat burning during aerobic activity, especially in untrained or inactive individuals.

An extensive analysis of 12 research found a link between increasing coffee consumption and a decreased risk of obesity, particularly in males.

A second study with 2,623 participants found a correlation between increased caffeine use and a better success rate for maintaining weight reduction.

Avoid adding a lot of cream or sugar to your coffee if you want to get the most health benefits.

Instead, have it without any milk or with a modest amount.

 Caffeine, which is present in coffee, may increase metabolism and fat-burning. According to studies, consuming plenty of caffeine may help you lose weight.

11. Incorporate Interval Training With High Intensity (HIIT)

High-intensity interval training (HIIT) is a type of exercise that keeps your heart rate up by alternating short bursts of action with long rest periods.

According to studies, HIIT is highly effective in increasing fat burning and fostering long

-term weight loss.

According to one study, performing HIIT three times per week for an average of 10 weeks dramatically decreased body fat mass and waist circumference.

HIIT also needed a 40% smaller time commitment for training than moderate-intensity continuous training, which includes exercises like jogging, rowing, and utilizing an elliptical machine.

Another study found that HIIT helped participants burn up to 30% more calories at the same time as other forms of exercise, including cycling or running.

Try walking and jogging or sprinting for 30 seconds at a time as a simple method to get started.

Additionally, you may alternate between movements like burpees, pushups, and squats with brief rest intervals in between.

Compared to other kinds of exercise, HIIT may improve fat burning and help you burn more calories quickly.

12. Include Probiotics In Your Meals

A form of helpful bacteria called probiotics can be discovered in your digestive system. It has been shown that these bacteria affect a wide range of functions, including immune and mental health.

Increasing your probiotic consumption through food or supplements will help you maintain your weight over the long run and increase your body's ability to burn fat.

Probiotic users had considerably bigger decreases in body weight, fat percentage, and BMI compared to those who took a placebo, according to a study of 15 research.

Another small trial found that

taking probiotic supplements
prevented fat and weight gain
in adults who followed a high-
fat, high-calorie diet.

Probiotics from the genus
Lactobacillus may help
people lose weight and fat in
particular ways depending on
the strain.

Taking pills is an easy and
practical approach to
consuming a daily
concentrated dosage of
probiotics.

You may also consume foods high in probiotics including kefir, tempeh, natto, kombucha, kimchi, and sauerkraut.

Increasing your diet of probiotic meals or using probiotic supplements may help you lose weight and lower your body fat percentage.

13. Examine Sporadic Fasting

A diet pattern is known as intermittent fasting cycles between periods of eating and fasting.

Although it might not be right for everyone, some studies suggest that it might improve both weight reduction and fat loss.

One study on intermittent fasting looked at alternate-day fasting, which involves alternating between days when you eat regularly and days when you don't.

This technique lowered body weight by up to 7% and body fat by up to 12 pounds over 3–12 weeks (5.5 kg).

Another small research found that when resistance training was paired with eating only eight hours a day, fat mass decreased and muscle mass was maintained.

Intermittent fasting comes in a variety of forms, such as

Eat Stop Eat, the Warrior Diet, the 16/8 technique, and the 5:2 diet.

Find a variant that matches your schedule, and don't be hesitant to try out different things to see what suits you the best.

14. Increase Your NEAT

Non-exercise activity training NEAT, also known as thermogenesis, refers to all the calories you burn while carrying out regular everyday activities like cleaning, vacuuming, putting out the garbage, playing the piano, fidgeting, and so on.

Even while this exercise may not seem like much, every little bit helps when it comes to losing body fat.

On the other hand, leading a sedentary lifestyle or spending too much time sitting down may promote fat storage.

Studies have shown that obesity and low NEAT levels are related. You risk losing it, though, if you relocate it.

Look for small adjustments you can make each day to add extra exercise to your schedule, such as using the stairs instead of the elevator, parking at the far end of the lot, or helping your neighbor bring their groceries inside.

15. Add Vinegar And Ferment To Your Diet

A healthy gut flora is a vital connection in safely decreasing body fat and keeping it off.

Naturally fermented foods

like pickles, sauerkraut, kimchi, kefir, and yogurt provide the substrates necessary for the growth of beneficial bacteria in the stomach.

16. Get Rid of Chemicals That Cause Fat

If fat reduction is your objective, examine your plastic for obesogens. You might not give much thought to the materials that your food is presented or wrapped in.

Obesogens are covert molecules that alter hormone levels, take over our metabolic processes, and even induce the body to store more fat.

Lowered growth hormone production, imbalanced cortisol levels, and higher insulin resistance are all effects of exposure.

These fat-producing chemicals are derived from substances that are present in plastics, food containers, nonstick cookware, pesticides, herbicides, artificial sweeteners, and hormones administered to cattle.

You may be familiar with Bisphenol-A (BPA), a synthetic estrogen used to harden plastic for products like water bottles and plastic food containers, as an example of an obesogen.

CHAPTER 4

Foods That Burn Fat and Rev Up Your Metabolism

Body fat may be decreased by eating specific foods. A person can gradually reduce weight and burn fat by including these fat-burning items in their diet. Eggs, almonds, and fatty fish are some examples of these fat-burning meals.

Foods that cause fat loss through enhancing metabolism, lowering appetite, or reducing total food intake may be referred to as "fat-burning foods."

Every meal increases metabolism. Chili peppers, for example, may have a greater effect on metabolism than other food kinds. Consuming these meals might help you lose weight.

Nuts, for example, have a longer-lasting effect on satiating hunger than other meals. These meals may aid in appetite regulation and decrease total calorie consumption, resulting in weight reduction.

In this book, we look at various meals that can help people lose weight because they burn fat. We also consider the most effective way to incorporate these items into the diet.

1. Berries

Berries are lower in sugar

than other fruits and are high in fiber (up to 9 grams per cup!) and antioxidants.

They are satisfying and healthy due to this combination. Nature's way of stating that everything wonderful comes in little packages is to eat berries.

These little fruits can serve whatever purpose you choose in your daily diet plan. They may be used as garnishes on your morning food or as an ingredient in nutritious smoothies.

You may eat them as snacks or prepare them into nutritious treats. Berries can be eaten raw, used in cooking, or even made into jams and marmalades.

They may take on whatever form you like and are flavor-packed. What else? You may eat them every day if you want since they are very nutritious! Antioxidants, which combat inflammation in the body and so lower the risk of cardiovascular disease and other health concerns, are abundant in berries.

2. Kefir

You have an overabundance of gut bacteria that cause desires if you've been following the conventional American diet, so you'll continue to eat that way.

Similar to kefir, these foods are naturally prebiotic, promoting the development of beneficial bacteria and improving how well your body breaks down food.

The drinkable yogurt didn't appeal to you? The same

principles apply to pickled vegetables, kimchi, and sauerkraut.

3. Avocados

Avocado is essentially a single-seeded fruit that is indigenous to Mexico, but it differs significantly from the usual produce aisles fare like blueberries and strawberries. It also has a ton of health advantages.

Your infatuation with avocado toast may be beneficial since a 2013 research found that habitual avocado eaters had reduced BMI and waist circumferences.

According to London, monounsaturated fats are also satisfying and heart-healthy, which means you won't be as tempted to munch on processed foods later in the day.

The 1 calorie in a raspberry is vastly outweighed by the 322 calories and 29.5 grams of fat in an avocado, which is 10 to 20 times more caloric than any other vegetable item. So it's reasonable to state that the avocado might theoretically be classified as a fruit rather than a fat.

Furthermore, studies claim that an avocado's 20 grams of monounsaturated fat per fruit are what makes it so unique and deserved its reputation as a healthy meal.

4. Salmon

Wild salmon is the only food that provides more of the omega-3 fatty acids that are good for the brain, heart, joints, and intestines.

It is also low in glycemic index, which means it doesn't cause insulin surges or belly fat accumulation. The key to maintaining thin is the balance of omega-3 and omega-6 fatty acids. Furthermore, salmon's delicious lipids make it harder to overeat.

5. Grapefruit

Research suggests that grapefruit and insulin have a

physiological connection to weight management.

According to the study, grapefruit's chemical composition lowers insulin levels and promotes weight reduction.

The significance of this connection is related to the hormone's role in weight regulation. While not its major purpose, insulin helps to control the metabolism of fat.

Grapefruit has certain chemicals that make your

body utilize insulin more effectively, lowering blood sugar levels and maybe increasing calorie burning. Maybe just avoid adding sugar before eating.

6. Walnuts

By modifying your insulin resistance, eating omega-3 fatty acids—which walnuts are packed with—activates fat -burning.

They are a crucial component of a low-glycemic diet, which, according to research, burns

300 more calories per day than a high-glycemic one.

7. Quinoa

This grain is popular for a reason. Quinoa is a terrific alternative to acid-forming grains like wheat and barley.

It gives you sustained energy and prevents bloating by feeding on the beneficial bacteria in your stomach.

8. Sardines

A nutritious diet that has

essential omega-3 fatty acids is fish. Salmon and other oily fish are especially rich in long-chain fatty acids, which are hard to get elsewhere.

Fish is a good source of protein. Protein in the diet helps quell hunger and is a key element in the weight reduction process.

Although not everyone like this fish, those who do are in for a tremendous treat.

Protein-rich foods like sardines assist to balance blood sugar, give you a feeling of fullness, and speed up your metabolism.

Second, they are a fantastic source of omega-3 fatty acids, which aid to improve mood in addition to strengthening the cardiovascular system.

Sardines have a low mercury content, and a high amount of omega-3 fatty acids, and are also high in choline and vitamin B.

Furthermore, high-quality

protein sources like sardines don't cause inflammation, unlike industrially produced or inhumanely bred animal products.

9. Kale

It's a good thing that this green is now available in every grocery shop and on most cuisines.

It is an alkaline meal that has a high fiber content that delays the release of glucose to reduce insulin spikes.

Additionally, it contains magnesium, which lowers stress hormones in the body, and invigorates iron.

Several qualities of kale can help with weight management.

First off, although having a relatively low-calorie count, it still has a considerable amount of bulk, which should make you feel satisfied.

Kale has a low energy density due to its low calorie and high water content. Numerous studies have demonstrated that eating a lot of meals with a low energy density can help with weight reduction.

A little quantity of fiber, an essential ingredient that has been associated with weight reduction, is also present in kale.

It seems reasonable that kale may be a good addition to a

weight reduction diet, even if
there are no trials specifically
assessing its impact on
weight loss.

10. Oil Of Olive

Instead of using butter or
cooking spray, coat your pan
with olive oil. It's packed with
omega-3 fatty acids, just like
fish oil, that supports the
health of your stomach, brain,
and other organs while
managing your appetite.

11. Artichokes From Jerusalem

These root vegetables often referred to as sunchokes, are rich in inulin, a prebiotic that encourages the growth of healthy bacteria in your body.

Having a hard time locating them? Asparagus and the majority of leafy greens are other high-fiber meals that are rich in inulin.

12. Hemp Seeds

Hemp has uses other than in

cosmetics. The seeds can also be healthy to sprinkle on salads and porridge.

Alpha-linolenic acids, a form of omega-3 fatty acid found in hemp seeds, have been shown in tests to increase metabolism.

13. Green Tea

Try it in place of coffee for your afternoon pick-me-up today.

According to research conducted on animals, the

active ingredients in green tea may facilitate this process by enhancing the actions of several hormones that promote fat burning, such as norepinephrine.

The primary antioxidant in tea, EGCG, may be able to stop an enzyme from degrading the norepinephrine hormone.

Norepinephrine production rises when this enzyme is blocked, boosting fat breakdown.

The natural compounds
EGCG and caffeine in green
tea may work together to
enhance health benefits.

Finally, extra fat is broken
down by your fat cell and
released into the circulation
where it may be used as
energy by cells like muscle
cells.

Green tea stimulates the
metabolism for many hours
by helping the thyroid
produce the hormone

thyroxine.

14. Brown Rice

This whole grain is naturally high in chromium, a substance that aids the body in controlling blood sugar levels. The outcome? decreasing the buildup of fat and insulin resistance.

15. Eggs

We have excellent news if you always start your day with eggs.

Although they have a bad reputation due to their high cholesterol level, eggs may be a component of a balanced diet.

According to research, eggs can even aid in weight loss since they provide a nutritious, high-protein breakfast option that keeps you satisfied.

According to the American Heart Association, eggs are full of vitamins, minerals, and other elements that are vital for good health (AHA). They contain a lot of cholesterol, but there isn't any solid proof

that consuming cholesterol
leads to high blood
cholesterol levels.

Eggs are a great source of
protein and can aid with
hunger management.
According to research
published in the journal
Nutrition Research, eating
eggs for breakfast helped
people better manage their
appetite and calorie
consumption throughout the
rest of the day.

What you need to know about

the nutritional advantages of eggs and how to include them in your weight-reduction plan is provided below.

Eggs are a particularly high-protein breakfast food that has been related to weight loss and the reduction of abdominal fat.

16. Steel-cut Oats

Steel-cut oats are a good choice if you want to consume healthy carbohydrates because they are known to speed up your metabolism.

Starch really "resists" being digested in the small intestine and prolongs your feeling of fullness.

17. Bananas

Given how much potassium bananas contain, starting your day with one might be beneficial for your metabolism.

Potassium aids in the body's regulation of the flow of minerals and fluids into and out of cells and may even boost basal metabolism, a measure of calories burnt when awake and at rest.

18. Heat Pepper

Ready to up the temperature? Adding a little spice to your life might significantly speed up your metabolism.

Peppers include a compound called capsaicin, which provides heat and promotes the burning of fat for weight reduction.

One research found that the heat from capsaicin in chilies caused participants to enhance their metabolism after eating for 30 minutes. The energy required for the chemical reaction during the metabolic process rises as a result of this heat.

Capsaicin, the naturally occurring substance in spicy peppers that causes the burning sensation, may aid with weight reduction due to its propensity to produce heat, burn calories, and break down fat, according to research.

19. Coffee And Palm Oil

Yes, olive oil is fantastic. However, coconut oil is also good for your metabolism, particularly when combined with palm oil. It has been demonstrated that consuming coconut and palm kernel oil in combination increases fat metabolism and energy expenditure.

20. Foods That Ferment

Probiotics are found in many

fermented foods, including miso, tempeh, and unsweetened plain Greek yogurt, and they can help regulate gastrointestinal health and reduce bloating.

21. Nuts

Nuts are incredibly nourishing. They are rich in protein and healthy fats, which both help to sate the appetite for extended periods.

Importantly, nuts may be

included in a healthy diet without causing weight gain.

For instance, research indicated that adding nuts to the diet for 12 weeks improved the quality of the diet without causing weight gain.

22. Yogurt

The nutritional value of yogurts might vary. The healthiest yogurt is plain yogurt, such as Greek-style yogurt. Numerous vitamins, minerals, and probiotics are included in it.

Other forms of protein found in yogurt include whey and casein.

According to a 2014 research published in the Nutrition Journal, consuming high-protein yogurt can help people manage their appetites, satisfy their hunger, and eat less overall.

23. Divided Peas

Peas are a good source of fiber, vitamins, and minerals. Additionally, they provide complex carbs, a wonderful source of energy.

Additionally, split peas include proteins that might quell appetite.

Dried pea protein reduces hunger more effectively than whey protein from milk.

24. Cayenne Peppers

The compound capsaicin, which is found in chili peppers, may help people lose weight.

Capsaicin may enhance fat burning and decrease appetite, according to a systematic study that was published in the journal Appetite in 2012. Weight loss may result from these factors.

25. Cocoa Butter

High levels of medium-chain triglycerides may be found in coconut oil. This particular kind of fat may offer several health advantages.

The Journal of the Academy of Nutrition and Dietetics published a meta-analysis in 2015 that suggested that medium-chain triglycerides could promote weight reduction. To corroborate the findings, additional research is necessary.

Medium-chain triglycerides

are thought by many experts
to boost metabolism and
decrease fat storage.

www.ingramcontent.com/pod-product-compliance
Lightning Source LLC
Chambersburg PA
CBHW061348250726

48657CB00004B/1383